Advances in Facial Cosmetic Surgery

Your Guide to Achieving the Best Long-Term Results

WILLIAM R. BURDEN
M.D., F.A.C.S.

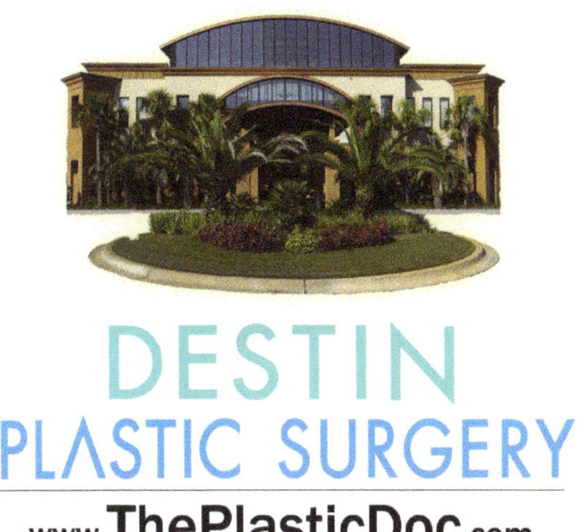

DESTIN
PLASTIC SURGERY
www.ThePlasticDoc.com

Published by William R. Burden, M.D., F.A.C.S., Destin, Florida.

ISBN: 978-0-578-71559-9

This book is not intended for use as a source of medical advice. The information in this book is intended to provide basic information on cosmetic facial surgery procedures and the subjects discussed. It is not intended to be comprehensive by any means. **This book is not intended to diagnose or to treat any medical conditions, or to replace the advice of the reader's physician(s).**

The reader should regularly consult a physician in matters related to his or her health, specifically with respect to any symptoms that may require diagnosis or medical attention. For diagnosis or treatment of any medical problems, consult your physician(s).

The author and publisher are not responsible or liable for any damages or negative consequences from any treatment, action, application or preparation to any person reading or following the information in this book.

While all attempts have been made to verify information provided in this publication, the author and publisher assume no responsibility for errors, omissions or contrary interpretation of the subject matter herein. Any perceived slights of specific persons or organizations are unintentional.

Any trademarks mentioned in this book are listed for reference purposed only and are the property of the respective trademark owners.

Table of Contents

Introduction

This book is intended to be an overview of cosmetic facial surgical procedures for men and women. I will be describing the most commonly performed facial surgical techniques including brow lift, eyelift surgery, and facelift procedures. It's important to understand that each patient is unique and ages differently. A consultation with a qualified plastic surgeon will help each individual patient decide which procedure or combination of procedures is the best solution for them. I believe the techniques described in this book provide the highest level of patient satisfaction when performed by an experienced, qualified plastic surgeon.

The Eyes

The eyes affect the expression of the face more than any other part of the face. We notice the eyes first when we engage another person in conversation and other social activities. The effects of aging reveal themselves first in the eyes. Three aspects that influence the appearance of the eyes are the position of the brow, the upper eyelids, and the lower eyelids. When the eyebrows have lowered, the eyes are partly closed, and the face assumes a concerned appearance. Excess skin on the upper eyelids gives the appearance of being tired and makes one look older. When the lower eyelids become puffy, they give the appearance of a poor night's sleep and can make one look old, tired, and sometimes angry. Fortunately, all three of these aspects can be surgically treated to improve the area around the eyes and restore a rested, youthful appearance.

The Face

There are several areas of the face and neck that change as people age. When we are young, a fat pad starts just over the cheekbone and ends around the middle of the cheek. As we age that fat falls downward, so it starts below the top of the cheekbone and ends over the mandible (or "jowl"), giving a heavier, droopy appearance. The platysma muscles on either side of the neck provide a smooth neck when we are young. These thin muscles separate in the middle with aging and bands on the neck appear. This is commonly referred to as a "waddle." The skin also loses elasticity as we age toward around age 50 for most people. It may be age 45 for some people, and 60 for others. Reduction in elasticity causes droopy, sagging skin with an increase in wrinkles on the face and neck. When performing facial rejuvenation or a facelift, most people need all three of these features addressed to restore the youthful appearance.

Minimally Invasive Brow Lift Research Using Fiber Optics

During my plastic surgery fellowship at the University of Florida, we were at a time when surgeons were transitioning from conventional surgeries to more advanced minimally invasive procedures using fiber optics and more sophisticated techniques. At that time, brow lifts typically required a large cut across the top of the scalp. A strip of skin and hair was removed, and a large scar remained after the surgery. Often this procedure resulted in numbness at the top of the head as sensory nerves in the scalp are usually divided during the surgery.

I had read about Dr. Rollin Daniels and the innovations he was applying to the brow lift procedure to make it much less invasive and to minimize the issues associated with the traditional brow lift. Although it was a very new technique, there was a lot of excitement in the cosmetic surgery community about this new, less invasive procedure. Dr. Daniels was very gracious in sharing the details of his endoscopic brow lift procedure with me and recommended the instruments needed for the surgery. I contacted the company that made the instruments and requested a loaner set to practice the procedure. I worked in the cadaver lab to familiarize myself with the instruments and improve my technique. I confidently performed the endoscopic brow lift on a patient. The outcome was excellent.

Every Tuesday surgeons in the fellowship program and professors presented interesting cases. At the same time I performed the endoscopic brow lift, one of our professors, who was not eager to learn the new procedure, performed a traditional brow lift on another patient. He presented his brow lift and it was a reasonable result. I would give it a B minus. I presented my case and the result was an A plus. This demonstration changed the minds of a lot of surgeons at the University of Florida when they observed the results of this procedure without having to cut out any hair. Over the years I have enhanced the procedure itself as well as the results.

Advances in Lower Eyelid Surgery

Traditional lower eyelid surgical procedures address the bagginess under the eyes, but unfortunately the result is not always great. While developing eyelid surgical techniques, I realized that we need to not only eliminate the bagginess of the eyelid, but to also lift the upper cheek. My procedure lifts the cheek pad off the cheekbone, elevates the pad, and repositions it on the cheekbone. The result is a shortened eyelid with a smooth transition between the eyelid and upper cheek, restoring a youthful appearance in the area beneath the eyes. Many cosmetic and oculoplastic surgeons are not trained to lift the upper cheek resulting often in suboptimal results.

The Composite Facelift

The skin loses its elasticity as people age. Facelifts were originally performed primarily by tightening the skin. The result with these early procedures was an apparent pulled, stretched appearance that most people associate with a bad facelift. I studied the work of Dr. Sam Hamra, a plastic surgeon in Dallas. Dr Hamra had developed the concept of the composite facelift. His idea was that the surgeon needs to not just tighten the skin, but to also move the underlying structures to achieve a natural looking appearance after the surgery. This involves elevating the cheek pad, tightening the muscles in the neck, and removing the inelastic skin. I've practiced this technique for many years and have developed advances to continually improve the procedure. One example is a special surgical maneuver to improve the neck contour, a critical area for the appearance of a woman. In recent years, the composite facelift concept has become more the standard of care for facelifts around the country.

Dr. Hamra also developed split-screen images showing the before picture on the left side and the after picture on the right side. When viewing the combined images, patients can get a good understanding of changes that can be made with facial surgery. These are a great tool to show potential patients what they can expect as a result of surgery. I've included some split-screen pictures of some of my actual patients later in the book.

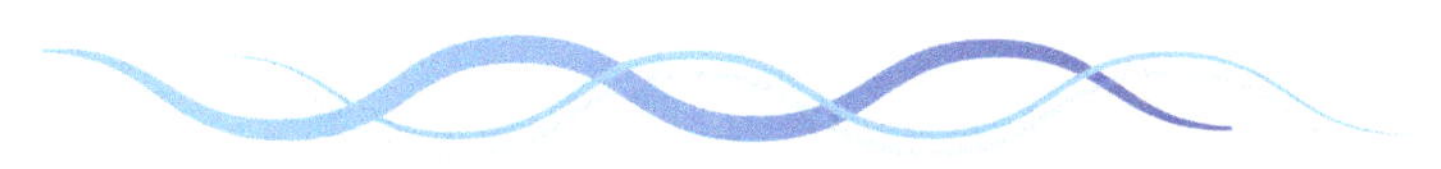

Questions & Answers (Q & A's)

Q: What are typical reasons that people consider having facial cosmetic surgical procedures?

A: Both men and women seeking facial cosmetic surgery are interested in looking better and regaining a more youthful appearance. As our society has become more fitness oriented, many men and women continue a very active lifestyle longer than they did in the past. Although they may be 65, 75, or even 85 years old, women and men can frequently be found on tennis courts, golf courses, or participating in other challenging activities. We often hear patients say, "I want to look as young as I feel." Executives, salespeople, and business owners want to look their best when meeting clients, in front of a camera, or on stage. Career is a motivation for some people, particularly for men who are extending their careers into their 60's and 70's.

Here are some areas that can be helped:

The Forehead and Brow

As we age, people develop deep furrows between their brows, the brow position lowers, and the skin beneath the brow begins to settle on the upper eyelid. Sometimes the eyelashes are covered!

These changes in anatomy gives the visual appearance of anger and fatigue. Patients remark they are frequently asked, "Are you tired?" or "Are you angry, because you look mad at something?" Patients go on to say, "I am well rested and in a good mood, but due to the wrinkles and loose skin around my eyes, I look tired and angry." That is when a browlift can be of benefit to their appearance and psyche.

The Lower Eyelid

Men or women also look tired, even when they're not, when they have baggy eyelids. They recognize they look tired when looking in the mirror. That mirror can be cruel when you see dark puffy areas under the eyes. Maybe their friends and colleagues frequently remark about how tired they look. They become wary of being repeatedly asked if they had a bad night, why they are so tired, or if they need a cup of coffee. A lower eyelid surgery (lower blepharoplasty) can dramatically improve the appearance of this area.

The Lower Face and Neck

Skin loses its elasticity as we age. The elasticity is generally good up until about 50 years, earlier for some people and later for others. Loss of elasticity causes the appearance of drooping, saggy skin with loss of jawline definition. The face also has an increase in wrinkles.

The neck contour and junction with the face may not be well defined. The skin and muscles of the neck become lax and a "waddle" begins to show in pictures and the mirror. Now is the time for a Facelift.

A brow lift might be right for you if:

- Your brows have become set lower and the eyes don't appear fully open
- You have deep furrows between the brows
- Your resting facial expression has the appearance of fatigue or anger.

Eyelid surgery might be right for you if:

- You constantly look tired, even when you're not
- You have dark, puffy areas below your eyes
- Other people frequently comment on how tired you look

A face lift might be right for you if:

- You have sagging or droopy skin on your face and neck
- You have increased wrinkles on your face or neck
- Your neck contour and jawline has become less well defined

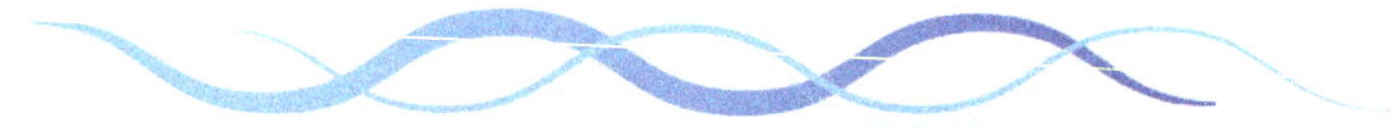

Q: Who are good candidates for cosmetic facial surgery?

A: Good candidates for cosmetic facial surgery are in good general overall health and cardiovascular fitness. We want to avoid any medical conditions that could cause excessive bleeding or poor healing. Smoking can affect the ability to heal. If you are a smoker you need to stop smoking at least a month in advance of surgery and continue to not smoke for a month or more after the surgery.

It's also very important to have reasonable expectations. During our consultation we'll show you before and after pictures of patients that have similar features to allow you to get an idea of how much improvement to expect. It's pretty rare that patients have unreasonable expectations, but I won't operate on someone who wants to look like a "movie star" or when the expectation is not possible, and the potential to achieve the desired outcome does not exist.

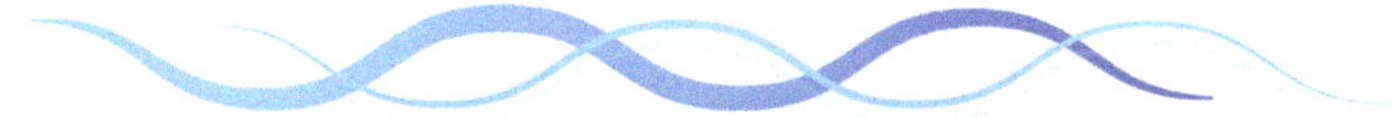

Q: At what age range are people typically seeking these procedures?

A: Women tend to start considering facial cosmetic procedures between the ages of forty-five and fifty-five. For men it's usually in the late fifties or early sixties—about ten to fifteen years later. Our society allows men to look a little older before they are considered to look aged. Men also get a little bit more of a pass on loose skin because they can camouflage it by growing a beard.

Q: How is an endoscopic brow lift performed?

A: As we age, the brows tend to become set lower on the forehead and the skin beneath the brows tends to fold over the eyelids. The eyes don't appear to be as open and the eyes take on an aged appearance. The forehead also develops deep furrows between the brows and even a fold over the bridge of the nose. These features give the visual illusion of anger. An endoscopic brow lift is a solution for most patients.

Unlike a traditional brow lift where a strip of hair is removed across the scalp of the forehead by making an incision from ear to ear, no hair is removed. The endoscopic browlift is performed internally through four small incisions about one centimeter in length in the scalp. The incisions are behind the hairline and heal so well, that rarely are you about to find them after they have healed. We use a very small scope with a camera that is inserted into the small incisions to guide the surgical procedure. With that guidance, we avoid injury to the nerves in the forehead while we are elevating the forehead and the brows. We also weaken the muscles in between the brows so that you cannot make as deep of a furrow and wrinkle. This softens the deep furrows in that area that gives a person a stern, angry appearance. The muscle isn't completely destroyed as that action may result in a blank expression on the face.

The hallmark of the procedure is when the scalp is released properly, it elevates and sticks back down to the skull in the right position. We ensure that by putting sutures internally that hold the scalp in position and until it adheres to the skull and other tissues. The adherence occurs within about seven to 10 days after surgery.

Q: How does your endoscopic browlift procedure provide better results than a traditional browlift still performed by many surgeons?

A: Our endoscopic browlift procedure is minimally invasive (small incisions with no hair removed), has a quicker recovery time, and allows patients to return to their normal lifestyle with less discomfort than the classic browlift. This is especially appealing to men and women who want to limit their time off from work. The endoscopic procedure also avoids nerve damage to the forehead scalp that can result in numbness on the top or back of the head.

The older, classic browlift (or forehead lift) is significantly more invasive. With the traditional procedure, a cut is made from ear-to-ear on the top of the head. A strip of skin and hair is removed, the scalp is pulled up, and then the scalp is sutured back together. This procedure can achieve a good cosmetic result, but there are disadvantages. A strip of hair is removed, and a scar may be visible on patients with thinning hair or short hair. As you get older, hair loss is not desirable. Also, the nerves under the scalp can be damaged with the older procedure, resulting in numbness on the top or back of the head.

Although the newer, endoscope browlift has been developed and improved over the past 25 years, about one-half of cosmetic surgeons who perform browlifts still practice the older procedure with all its disadvantages.

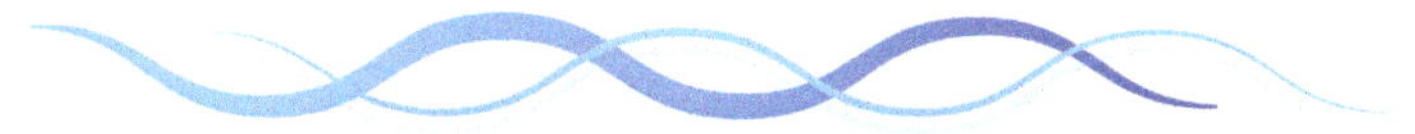

Q: Some patients may seek, or their physician may suggest, upper eyelid surgery. If upper eyelid surgery is indicated, why is it important to have a brow lift prior to upper eyelid surgery?

A: Some people have upper eyelids that appear droopy or puffy and they appear tired and aged. They may have been told that upper eyelid surgery is a solution to improve the puffiness. Unfortunately, the wrong procedure is often performed. A brow lift would have been the appropriate procedure and upper eyelid surgery should only be done if excess skin or bulging of the upper eyelid fat is apparent after the brow lift.

The eyebrow position acts as the scaffold on which the upper eyelid is "hung." The brow should be placed in its proper position first.

In explaining the brow lift concept to patients, I use the analogy of a window, curtain, and curtain rod. Think of the eye as a "window," the upper eyelid as the "curtain," and the brow as the "curtain rod." If the curtain rod is partway down the window, and the curtain begins to puddle on the floor, you wouldn't cut off the curtain. You would raise the curtain rod to the proper position and then adjust the curtain.

This is the concept of structural rejuvenation area around the eye:

First- elevate the outer brow correcting the upper eyelid hooding;
Second- improve the fold and furrows between the brows;
Third- remove the bags beneath the eyes and elevate the cheek pad.

Restoring the facial harmony prevents the operated-on appearance.

By looking carefully at the skin between your eyebrow and your upper eyelid, you will notice that the skin immediately below the brow is thick and of a different color and texture than the skin covering the eyelid. The eyelid skin is usually darker and thinner and much more supple. It's not appropriate to resect this upper eyelid skin when the brow is low and needs to be elevated. That upper eyelid skin is unique on the human body and cannot be replaced once removed. The eyebrow position acts as the scaffold on which the upper eyelid is based. The brow should be placed in its proper position first. After that, if extra skin or bulging of the upper eyelid fat is apparent, upper eyelid surgery can be performed safely.

We are frequently consulted by patients for improvement of their upper eyelid appearance after they have had upper eyelid surgery. They may have realized they need a brow lift; however, a brow lift cannot be performed because skin removed from the previous upper eyelid surgery would prevent them from being able to close their eye when the brow is elevated to the proper position.

Q: How is lower eyelid surgery performed and are there any special enhancements you use when performing the procedure?

A: Although a few wrinkles around the eyes add expression to a person's appearance, the development of dark circles, droopy lower eyelids, or bags under the eyes convey an undesirable fatigued appearance. The upper cheek pads also fall and begin to droop as we age. This contributes to the eyelids taking on an elongated and puffy appearance. In the past surgeons performing this procedure only addressed the eyelid bags. They did not address the upper cheek pad droop. This resulted in a hollowed out, elongated appearing lower eyelid. This is a suboptimal procedure and the resulting appearance is not as good as it could be.

The procedure I perform addresses the upper cheek pad droop, as well as, the baggy eyelid. I've developed a very technically exacting procedure to dissect the cheek pad off the cheekbone, elevate it, and reposition it to the proper place on the bone. The process takes experience and an eye for the proper positioning. The result is an elevated cheek pad, a shortened eyelid, and a smooth transition zone where the upper cheek meets the lower eyelid. This "contouring" of the lower eyelid avoids the pulled tight appearance that patients want to avoid.

Q: How is the composite facelift procedure performed?

A: Another result of ageing is the loss of skin elasticity, resulting in the appearance of saggy skin. The fat pad over the cheekbone falls downward, giving a droopy appearance. We also usually experience an increase in wrinkles in the face and neck and less definition of the neck and chin as the muscles in the neck separate. The composite facelift addresses all these areas and may be combined with a brow lift and eyelid surgery for a comprehensive rejuvenation of the face and neck to restore a youthful appearance.

A key principle of the composite facelift is that we don't merely remove and stretch excess skin that has lost its elasticity, but we also reposition underlying structures in the face and neck. We elevate the cheek pad, restoring it to the same position it was in during youth. We also tighten the muscles in the neck. Fat may be removed from some areas and replaced in areas of deficit. The skin is then redraped over the new underlying frame and any excess skin is removed. The result is a much less pulled or stretched appearance and the results of the facelift are retained for a longer period of time.

Every patient is unique, and there is some variation among patients in areas of the face and neck, so we individualize the procedure for each patient. Incisions are made in front of the ear, extending behind the ear lobe, and into the scalp behind the ear. These incisions heal well after surgery and very rarely are noticed after recovery. Raising the cheek pad makes a smooth transition from eyelid to cheek, regaining the appearance of youth in this area. The neck contour is critical for a woman's appearance and I use a special technique that yields a smooth, well-defined neck and chin. There are some differences in the way a facelift is performed between men and women to retain masculine and feminine characteristics.

Q: Why do the facelift procedures you have developed provide a superior result to the traditional "nip and tuck?"

A: For more than fifty years plastic surgeons used a "nip and tuck" philosophy to tighten excess skin that had lost its elasticity. Excess skin was excised ("nipped") and the incision was closed ("tucked"). The results were generally good; however, the early result often gave the patient a pulled or stretched appearance. Skin assumes the shape of the underlying facial structures and since those structures were not surgically altered, the tightly pulled skin relaxed after the facelift. As a result, the underlying aged face began to "show through" the skin. Over many years we have developed and improved the facelift procedure as explained earlier. These improvements result in a much less stretched appearance and the results will last for a longer period of time.

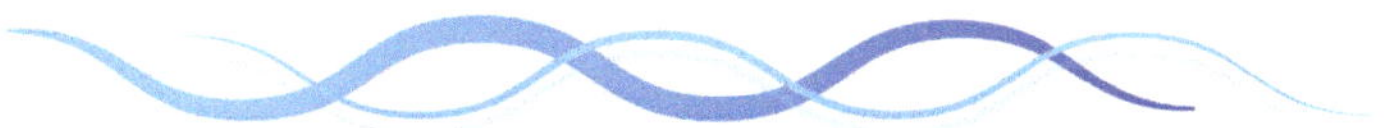

Q: There are some facelift procedures commonly advertised as minimally invasive and quick fixes. Will these procedures provide a good result?

A: Many surgical procedures with tradenames are commonly advertised on TV, radio, or in other media. Some of them are marketed as quick fixes and an alternative to a traditional surgical facelift. These may just be gimmicks to get people in the office.

Unfortunately, I see a significant number of people who had these advertised procedures performed with suboptimal results. They needed a much more extensive procedure and therefore the results they wanted were not realized.

Some women come in for a consultation after seeing an advertisement for the quick fixes and ask for a very specific named procedure. Often, that is not the right solution for them. Many times, the facial aging is way beyond what one of these quick fixes can address. The patient may really need a conventional facelift with removal of excess skin, the cheek pad lifted, and underlying muscle tightening.

During a consultation we will review some of our patients' before and after pictures and compare to the ones most similar to your face and condition and discuss the surgical approach that was needed to achieve the desired outcome.

Q: If a patient has "crow's feet" around the eyes, will a facelift solve that condition?

A: "Crow's feet" around the sides of the eyes cannot be solved with a facelift or other surgical procedures. There are non-surgical treatments that can help in the early stages of the aging process, such as BOTOX® Cosmetic, injectable fillers like Restylane® and JUVEDERM® Injectable Gel. These treatments are not permanent but "crow's feet" can be softened and often eliminated with these treatments. Many men prefer BOTOX injections because they provide subtler results.

Q: If a patient needs a facelift, browlift, and eyelid surgery, would the procedures typically all be done at the same time?

A: The eyes age first for most people and the lower face second. Often, we will perform a facial surgery in stages with a brow lift and eyelid surgery in a patient's forties and then a facelift later when they enter their fifties.

The most common situation, however, is to perform all the procedures at one time to comprehensively rejuvenate the face and neck. People are very busy with families, physical activities, and work, and they don't want to take three or four weeks off from life multiple times. There is only one recovery period by completing all of them at the same time.

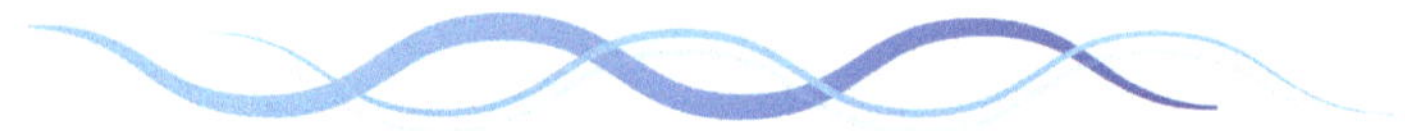

Q: Men and women generally have different facial characteristics. How does facial surgery typically differ between males and females?

A: Certain positions of anatomical features have a more masculine appearance or feminine appearance. A prime example is the brow. A woman's brow looks best when it's arched and sits approximately one finger breadth above the upper rim of the eye socket. A man's brow should sit right on that rim. If you elevate a man's brow to the position of a woman's brow, the new brow position will feminize his appearance or make him look boyish.

Likewise, a tight, distinct jaw line is a desirable feature for a female. When performing a facelift on a man we don't want to pull the jaw line too tight because that will result in an undesirable appearance on a man.

Even though the surgical procedures may be the same, these nuances need to be considered when planning for and doing the procedure. Adjustments are made in the skin tension, elevations, and where the fixation sutures are placed so a male is not feminized. Probably the most feared consequence for a facelift on a man is a feminized look or with the skin appearing overly pulled and stretched.

Q: What is the recovery like after facial cosmetic surgery?

A: The recovery time for a facelift in general, is about three to four weeks, and about two to three weeks for a brow lift or eyelid surgery. There will be some bruising and swelling in the areas treated for about two weeks, so it may be the third week after surgery where you feel comfortable going out in public. Pain is rarely mentioned by the patients, although patients will take a narcotic pain reliever for the first couple of days. After that, a narcotic may be needed to help sleep at night for a few additional days. Most patients feel fine after just three or four days, although they look pretty rough due to the bruising and swelling. Some facelift patients will feel a little tightness in the neck during the first week of recovery.

We don't want patients engaging in heavy physical activity for approximately four to six weeks depending on how much surgery they've had. We want to avoid increasing the blood pressure which could cause bleeding or additional swelling. After six weeks, they can return to any strenuous activities they prefer. Most patients feel comfortable with light exercise and walking at approximately two weeks. In general, three to six weeks is adequate for recovery to allow returning to your normal social activities.

If you have a job where you have a lot of face time with clients or you have to be out in public, you're going to need to take off three or four weeks where you're not visible, so you don't feel so self-conscious. On the other hand, if you have a job you can do in the back office or you can do from home, where you'll be on the phone or on a computer, you'll feel good enough to resume your work in three or four days.

The largest obstacle with facial surgery is having the time where you can be out of the public eye for three to four weeks. If you're getting prepared for a family event like a wedding, reunion, or other special event, plan to have the surgery three to six months in advance, so you will look your best at the event and in photographs.

Q: Will there be visible scars after facial cosmetic surgery?

A: It is extremely rare that a scar needs to be revised after I have performed facial surgery. The incisions made for a brow lift are well hidden behind the hair line, so any resulting minor scarring will not be seen. The incisions made for lower eyelid surgery are right under the eyelash line and they heal very well. A facelift requires larger incisions than the other procedures, around the ears and under the chin, but this area also heals very well and very rarely will a scar be easily noticed.

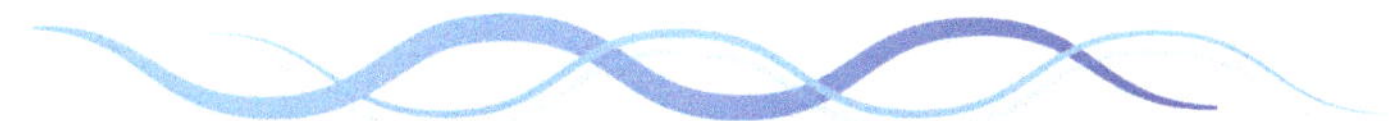

Q: How long will the results last for these procedures?

A: A brow lift generally will last for ten to fifteen years. Lower eyelid surgery normally lasts about fifteen years. A facelift will typically last for about seven to ten years. The surgery improves the structure of the face and the tightness of the skin. You want to look better, so you need to take care of the skin as well. If you damage your skin by smoking or not using sunscreens, then it's defeating the purpose of having the procedure which improved the shape of the face.

Light chemical peels or even heavier peels and BOTOX all help maintain the appearance of the skin, diminish the wrinkles, and help prolong the result of a facelift and enhance the appearance of the face. I recommend patients receive BOTOX around the eyes to address crow's feet and the forehead to help with wrinkles in that area. BOTOX relaxes the muscles, so they don't contract as much, reducing wrinkles. Fillers can also be placed to help improve the appearance of wrinkles around the mouth and to enhance the appearance of the lips. A chemical peel or laser resurfacing every three or four years will also help improve the appearance of the skin.

Q: What are the risks of facial surgery?

A: With any surgery, there is a risk of infection, but that's very low. Our surgeries are performed in an operating room with a very sterile environment. The main concern with facial surgery is bleeding. Patients need to have their blood pressure under control and not use medicines like aspirin, Advil, Aleve or supplements that can cause bleeding immediately before surgery or during the post-surgery recovery period.

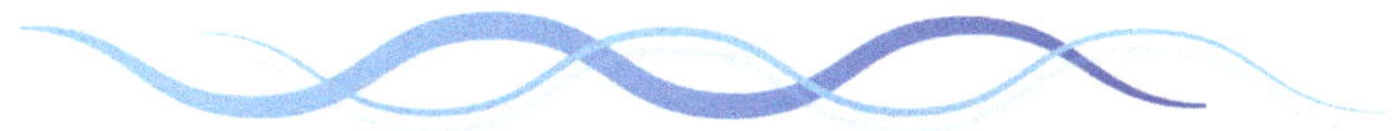

Q: How should a qualified surgeon be chosen to perform facial cosmetic surgery?

A: One good starting point is to get referrals from friends who have had good results with facial surgery. You might also want to get referrals from physicians. Not all plastic surgeons perform a lot of facelifts, so a good reputation and extensive experience performing facelifts and other facial surgery should be critical factors considered when selecting a surgeon. Ask to see pictures of results of actual patients and testimonials from actual patients. I've been developing, enhancing, and performing advanced facial surgical techniques for over twenty-five years. Very few surgeons have a similar level of expertise.

A good experience for the patient starts with good communications and rapport with your surgeon. Your surgeon should provide a thorough understanding of the procedure you are seeking and answer all your questions. Make sure that you sense that you and your surgeon have a compatible personality and philosophy during your consultation.

Finally, make sure that your surgeon is Board Certified by the American Board of Plastic Surgeons.

Before and After Pictures

On the following pages are **<u>actual</u>** before and after photos of four of Dr. Burden's facial cosmetic surgery procedure patients.

Readers can see an extensive gallery of Dr. Burden's patients' before and after photos from various procedures by visiting:

https://www.ThePlasticDoc.com

Patient 1

BEFORE
FEATURES
OF AGING
Flattened
Brow Arch
Loss of
Upper Face
Fullness
Jowls
loss of Definition
AFTER
YOUTHFUL
FEATURES
Arched Brow
Upper
Face
Fullness
Defined
Jaw Line

BEFORE
AFTER
Flat
Brow
Jowls
Neck
Bands
Arched
Brow
Defined
Jawline
Smooth
Neck

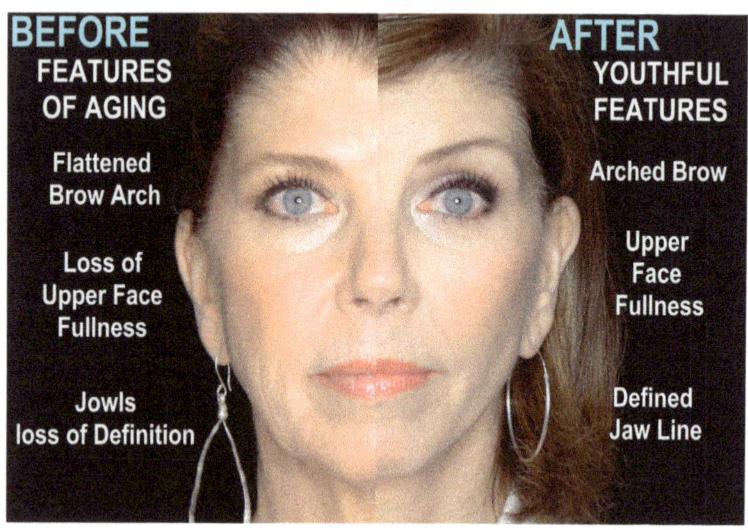

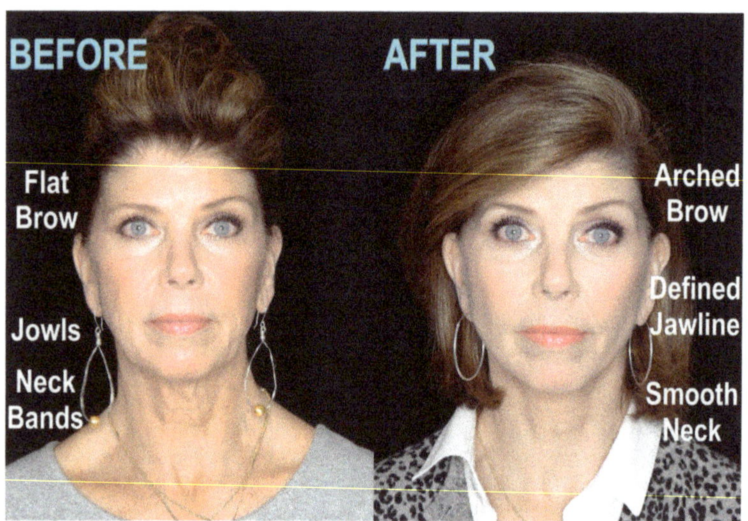

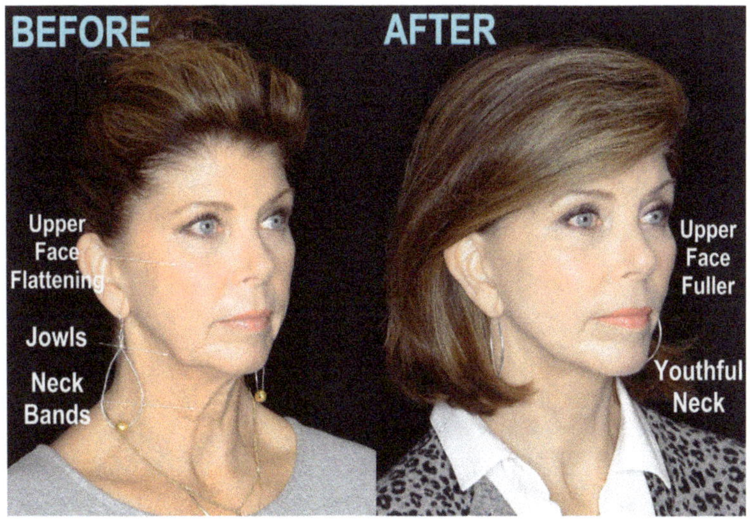
BEFORE
AFTER
Upper
Face
Flattening
Jowls
Neck
Bands
Upper
Face
Fuller
Youthful
Neck

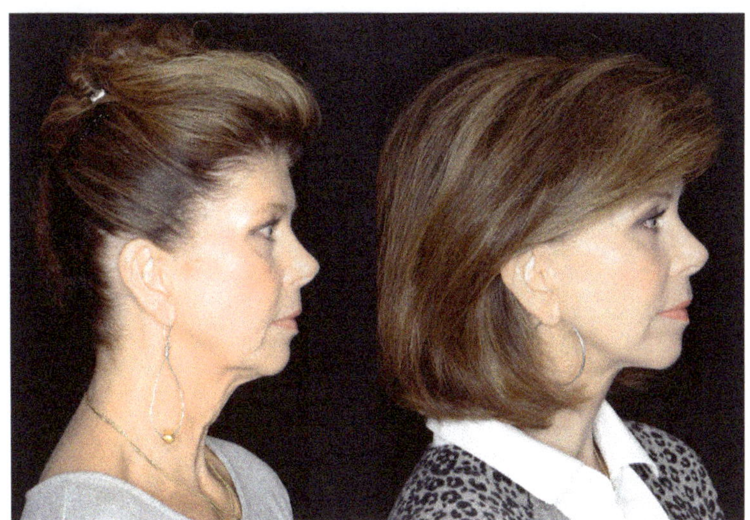

Patient 2

BEFORE
AFTER
Brow Droop
Full
Lower Face
Poorly Defined
Neck
Arched Brow
Full
Upper Face
Defined
Neck

BEFORE
AFTER

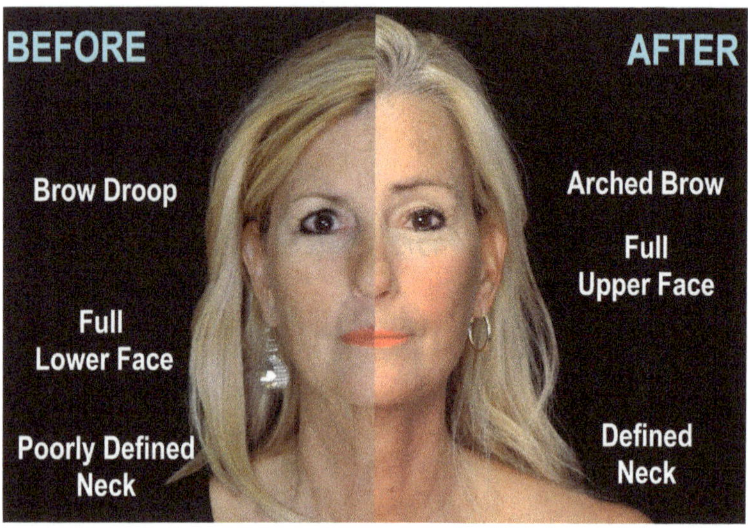

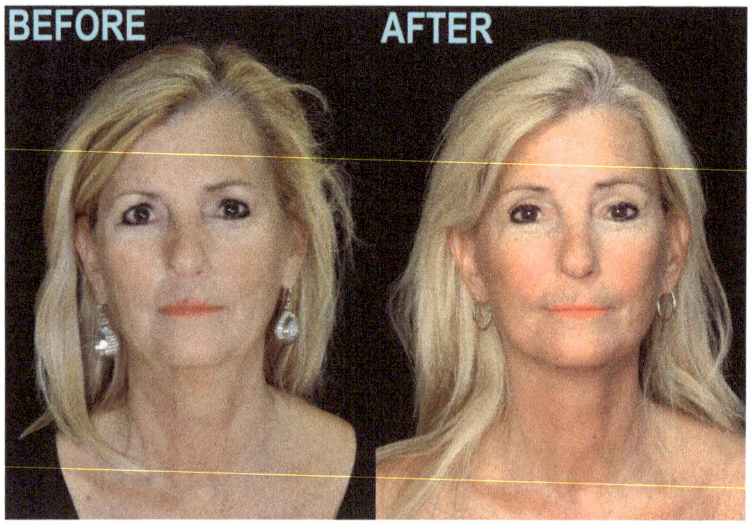

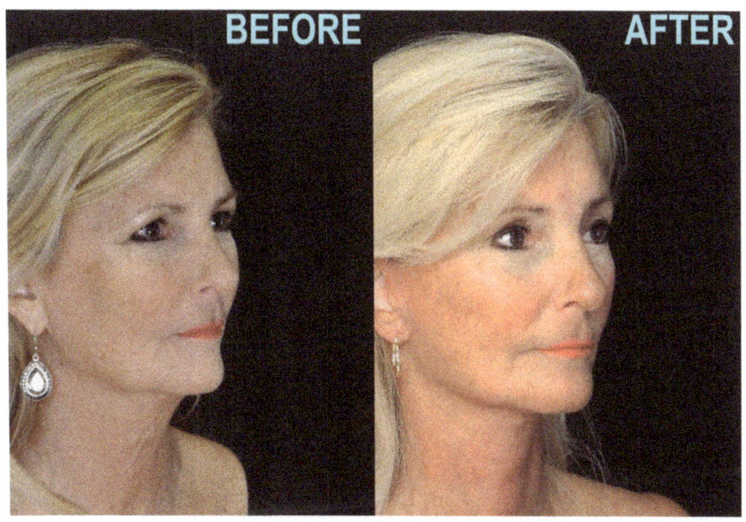
BEFORE
AFTER

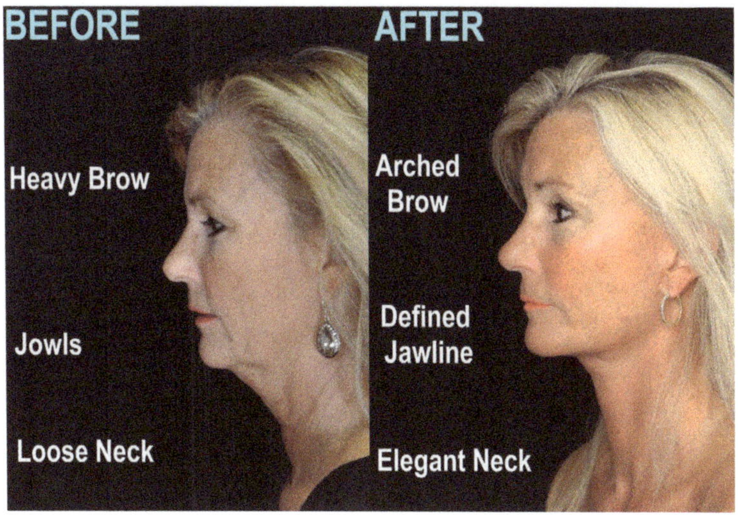
BEFORE
Heavy Brow
Jowls
Loose Neck
AFTER
Arched Brow
Defined Jawline
Elegant Neck

Patient 3

BEFORE
FEATURES OF
AN AGING FACE
Elongated
Lower Eyelid
Lower Face Fullness
Jowling
AFTER
FEATURES OF A
YOUTHFUL FACE
Youthful
Eyelid/Cheek
Junction
Upper Face Fullness
Defined Jawline

BEFORE
Heavy Brow
Bags Beneath
Eyes
Full
Lower Face
AFTER
Nicely Arched
Brow
Youthful
Lower Eyelid
Full
Upper Face

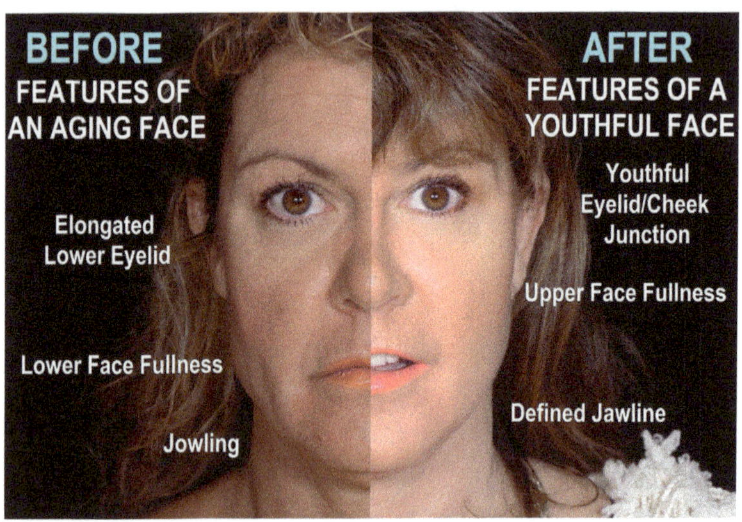

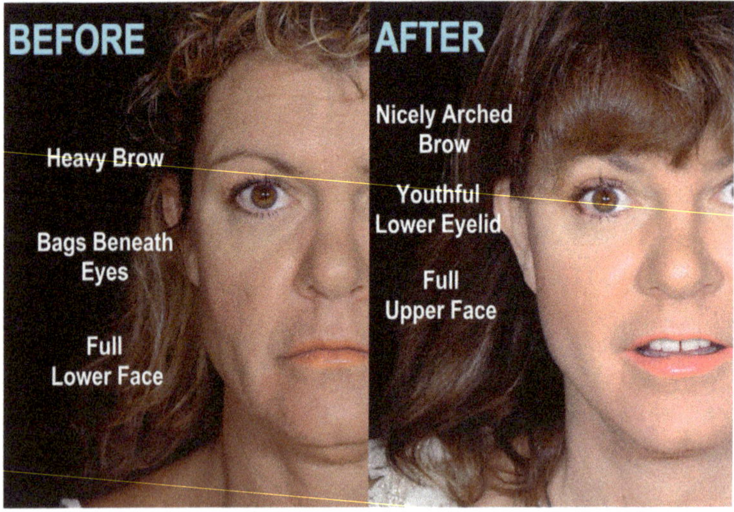

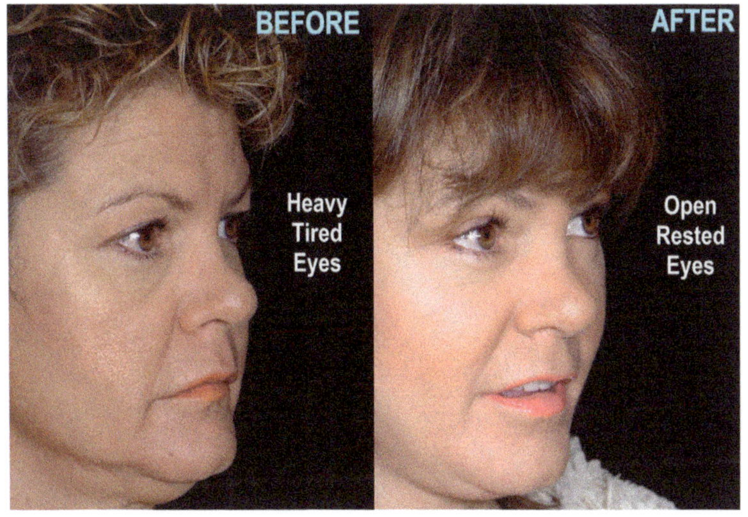
BEFORE
Heavy
Tired
Eyes
AFTER
Open
Rested
Eyes

Patient 4

BEFORE
Heavy Brow
Eyelid Bags
Jowls
AFTER
Arched Eyebrow
Youthful Lower Eyelid
Defined Jawline

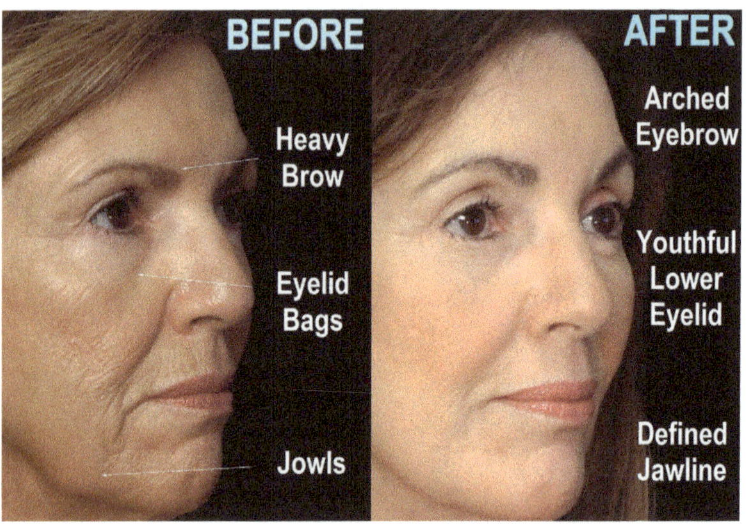

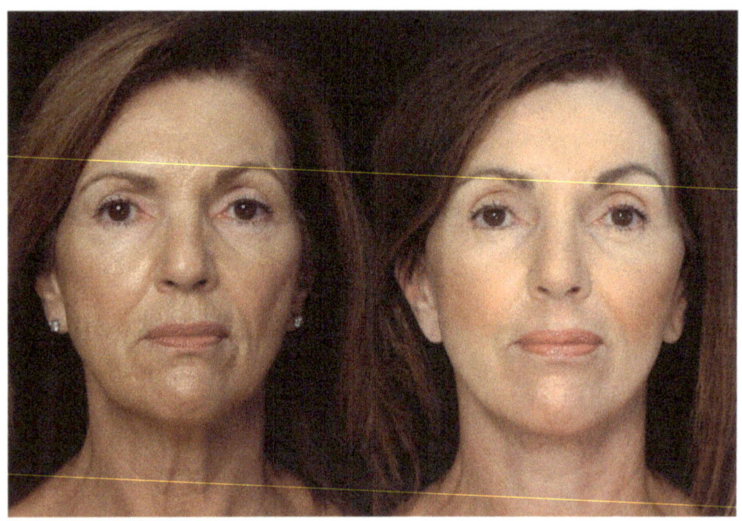

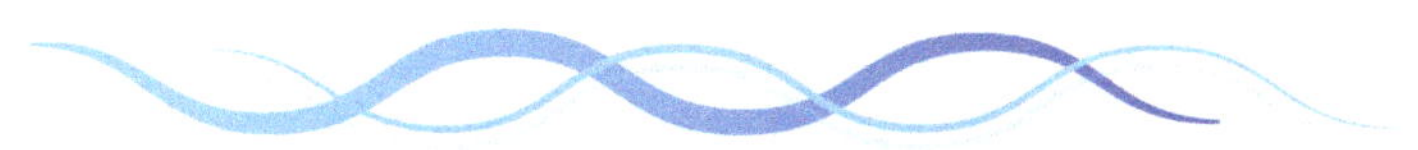

What Patients Are Saying

"Dr. Burden,

I had recovered from surgery and was out at a social function. I had just returned from Florida. Several of the ladies remarked on how I had returned from my vacation looking fabulous. I looked so good, but didn't look operated upon. No one suspected that I'd had surgery. Dr. Burden delivered exactly what I wanted!"

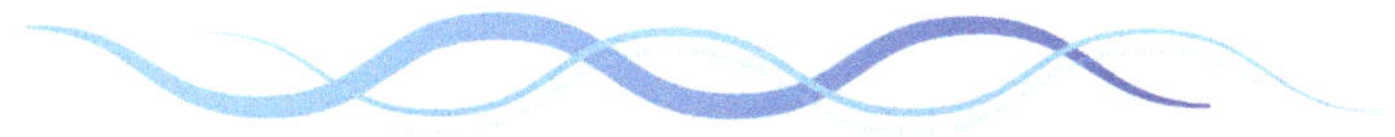

"Dr. Burden,

You made this a great year for me and I look forward to you working more magic on me!"

D.W., Panama City Beach, FL

"Dear Dr. Burden,

I want to thank you so much for a wonderful job that you did for me. My lower eyelids and the lipo. My daughter is very happy with her lipo too. You will never be replaced! You are the best."

I.C., Fort Walton Beach, FL.

"Dear Dr. Burden,

A quick note to say thank you for Destin Plastic Surgery and the wonderful people there. Thank you for your smile and kindness in the midst of all you do. Thank you for the results of my surgery. I'm excited about all the changes. I'm happy I had this surgery at the place and time and very grateful to have had you as my surgeon."

G.E., Crestview, FL

"Dr. Burden,

I can't begin to describe how my life has changed since my surgery. The surgery has truly changed my life. My family and friends love my new look and I am confident and pleased with my appearance. I am no longer hesitant to engage in social activities and am sometimes overwhelmed at how well I am received. My only regret is that I didn't make the decision to have the surgery years before. It is difficult to articulate how fortunate and blessed I feel as a result of the care you and your staff provided. The pre-counseling was informative and precise. Your staff was always available to answer my questions, they called my home to check on me and the flowers were a really sweet gesture as well. People often ask me why I am so happy and I can't wait to tell them of the miracle I received!"

C.J., Freeport, FL

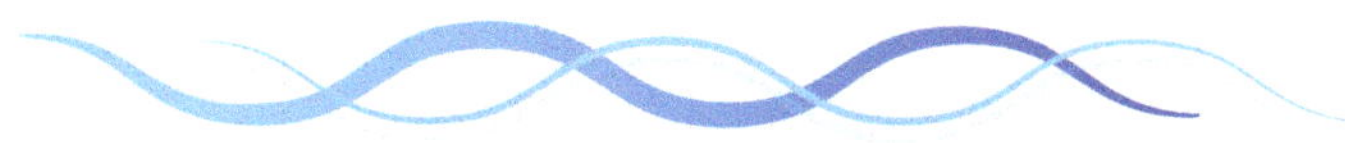

"Thank you Dr. Burden for excellent communication skills. I was so impressed with the amount of time you spent with me during the consultation. All of my questions were answered

without making me feel rushed through the office. I see now why Destin Plastic Surgery has an excellent reputation."

BP, New Orleans, LA

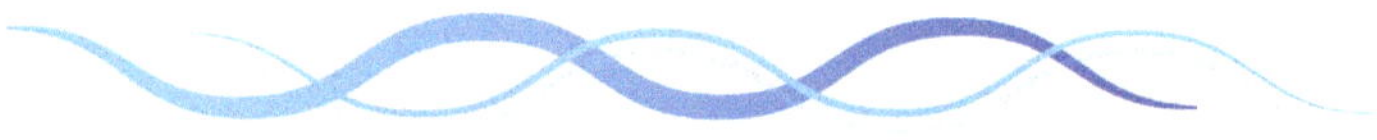

"Dr. Burden and Staff,

I wanted to tell you all thank you for the wonderful care I received. You truly changed my life!"

S.M., Pensacola, FL

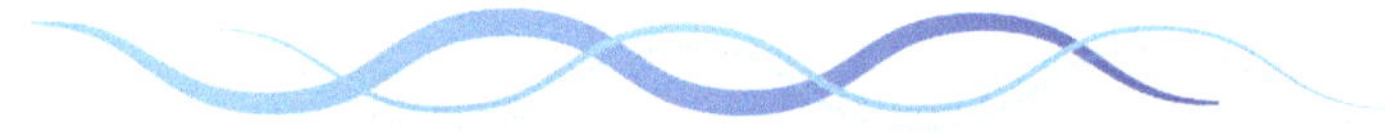

"Thanks to The Best Plastic Surgery Team in the World!

Dr. Burden and Staff,

Thanks for the beautiful yellow roses you sent me after my surgery. Thanks for being there for me and the outstanding service you always give with a smile. Each of you always made me feel so special and to think you do this with each of your patients/ clients. Thanks."

M.M., Navarre, FL

"Dr. Burden, Bill, Joan, and all the staff at the desk and in the operating room. I don't just smile I say, "Destin Plastic Surgery is the place to go!!" You are the best. Thank you!"

M.S., Mary Esther, FL

"Dr Burden,

I want to personally thank you and your staff for your kindness and wonderful care! I do appreciate all that you have done! Very Respectfully,"

L.P., Huntsville, AL

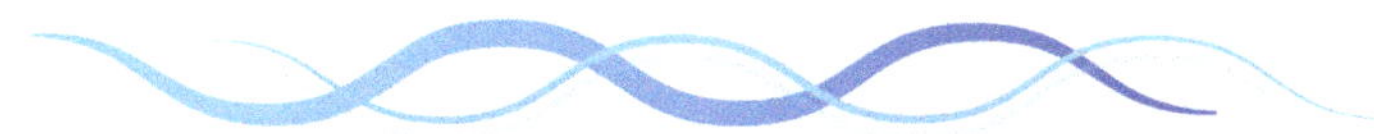

"Dr Burden,

Thank you for making my dreams come true!"

P.N., FWB, FL

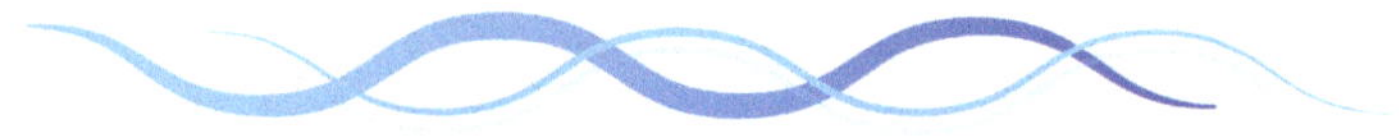

"Dr. Burden,

I just wanted to take the time *to thank you for the awesome experience I had with you and your staff when I had my* breast augmentation. *As a registered nurse, I know a little bit about what to expect with the* health *care system, but you and your* office *made my experience beyond words. Not only am I very happy with the surgical results, the whole experience made me feel very positive. It has been eighteen months since my final surgery and the final results are great! Thanks again."*

TC, Cantonment, FL

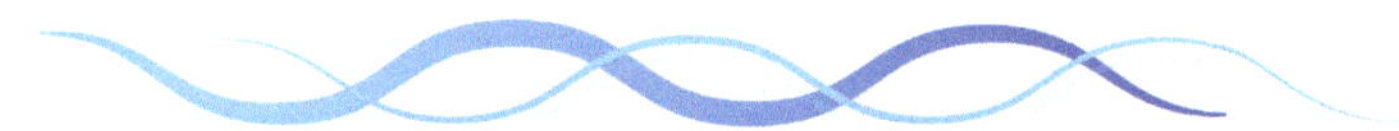

"Dear Dr. Burden and Staff,

I can tell already what a beautiful job you have done. It is the first time since my cancer surgery five years ago that I like my face. You are an incredible man Dr. Burden. You will never know what this means to me. Many thanks and God bless you. Love."

I.L.

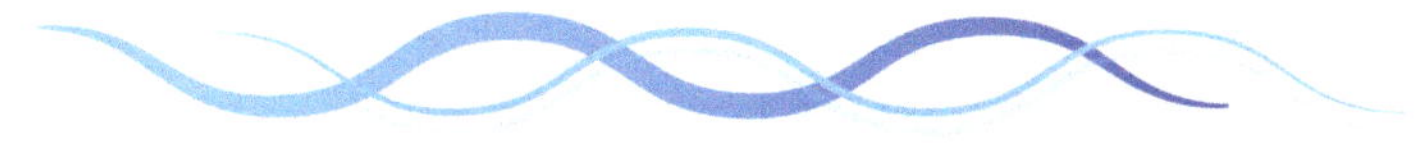

"Dear Dr. Burden and Staff,

Thank you so much! Your staff of the surgery center was awesome and I felt I had the very best of care! I am so happy with my result and feeling great just 24 hours after surgery. Thank you all again! May God richly bless each one of you!"

N.K.

"You really make me feel appreciated and that means so much to me. Your gift was more than generous and I thank you so much. You are enjoyable to work with, also your staff. Thanks."

D.

"Team work makes everything come together. Thanks to everyone of your team Dr. Burden, for making something very special happen for my husband and I. The professionalism with

which your organization functioned was exceptional. Thanks to all of them and especially you and your staff. You've helped put a smile back on my face."

L. *and* L. S.

About the Author

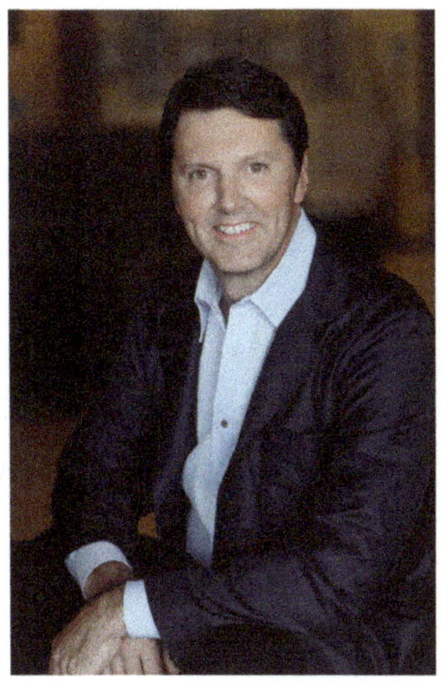

William R. Burden, M.D., F.A.C.S., is a Board Certified Plastic Surgeon, a Fellow of the American College of Surgeons and a member of the American Society of Plastic Surgeons. He is the founder and CEO of Destin Plastic Surgery in Destin, Florida, one of the Southeast's most recognized cosmetic facilities. He is also the founder of the Destin Surgery Center, housed in the same building.

While in high school, Dr. Burden took anatomy classes offered at the Medical College of Virginia on the weekends. He also took classes in Medical Genetics and Computer programming. Because of high PSAT and SAT scores, he was selected to attend college classes prior to graduating from high school at Virginia Tech.

Dr. Burden received his Bachelor of Science in Biochemistry and Biology with a minor in Chemistry and emphasis in Computer Science from Virginia Tech. He received his Medical Degree from the Medical College of Virginia. While at Virginia Tech, he was involved in genetics research. At the Medical College of Virginia, he was involved in Vitamin A research and its role in cancer prevention.

Dr. Burden completed his residency in General Surgery at Louisiana State University School of Medicine. While there, he authored several papers and was involved in vascular surgery research involving carotid artery grafting and spinal cord research involving anoxic injury to the spine.

While in his fellowship in Plastic Surgery at the University of Florida, Dr. Burden worked with his professors to introduce endoscopic techniques in breast and facial surgery and specialized microvascular techniques (DIEP Flaps) for breast and body reconstruction.

During his fellowship at the University of Florida, Dr. Burden was one of the pioneers in researching the use of endoscopic or fiber optic technology for plastic surgery. He saw the potential for use of this new technology to improve results in facial cosmetic surgery and to enable accurate placement of breast implants using an incision in the underarm area instead of on the breast.

Dr. Burden's vision was to perfect a procedure using the latest technology that would provide the best results in terms of breast augmentation without leaving a visible scar on the breast. Although some breast augmentations had been done by plastic surgeons using an incision in the armpit prior to this time, the ability to accurately dissect and place the implants was a limiting factor in the use of this technique. During the course of his fellowship, Dr. Burden and the team he was working with were successful in achieving his vision.

When Dr. Burden entered private practice, he offered the transaxillary approach, with the incision in the armpit along with the more traditional approaches to breast augmentation. Even though all of the approaches to breast augmentation can provide good results in terms of breast volume and shape, over time, he found that the highest patient satisfaction level was achieved when the patient had no scar on the breast.

Dr. Burden is known nationally and internationally for the No Scar on the Breast procedure. He has been performing the No Scar on the Breast procedure for over twenty years and has completed thousands of No Scar on the Breast surgeries.

Women travel from across the country and from around the world to have their procedures performed by Dr. Burden. Among his patients are Miss USA and Miss America contestants, country music performers and bathing suit models, to mention a few. In addition to breast augmentation, Dr. Burden performs a full range of cosmetic and reconstructive surgical procedures on the face and body. He has appeared on news reports for his expertise with the Brazilian Butt Lift, facelifts, and eyelid surgery.

Dr. Burden has been on the Mentor Corporation advisory panel for both breast augmentation and breast reconstruction. He is also on the Allergan Corporation advisory panel for new technology in breast augmentation and for their facial aesthetics and injectables products. He is a member of the Allergan Speaker Bureau and instructs and educates other physicians, nurses, and medical personnel on facial aesthetic treatments. In addition, he has participated in the national study for the reintroduction of the silicone gel implant.

Dr. Burden has been added to a panel of surgeons advising plastic surgeons on the use of the REVOLVE system to improve the results of fat grafting. The surgeons on this panel are experienced with fat grafting to enhance the appearance on areas of the body including the face, breasts, buttocks, hands, and other areas needing contouring.

Dr. Burden's surgeries are conducted at the Destin Surgery Center, co-located with Destin Plastic Surgery. The center is fully accredited by the Accreditation Association for Ambulatory Health Care and was ranked as one of the best hospitals by *US News and World Report.* Over 30,000 procedures have been performed at this facility. A full-time attending anesthesiologist is the Medical Director of Destin Surgery Center.

For More Information

For more information about Dr. William Burden, facial cosmetic surgery, and other cosmetic surgical procedures, visit:

https://www.ThePlasticDoc.com

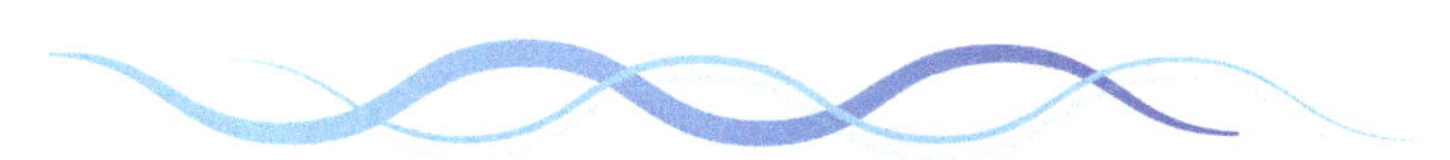

Contact Information

Destin Plastic Surgery
The Grant Building
4485 Furling Lane
Destin, Florida 32541

Phone: (850) 654-1194
Toll-free: (866) ENHANCE (364-2623)

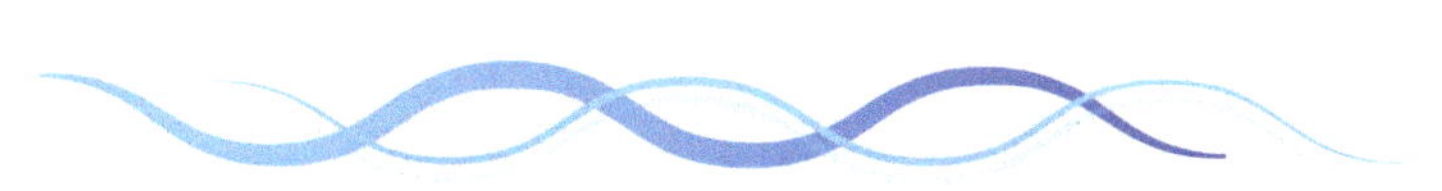

Glossary

Brow Lift: A cosmetic surgical procedure, also known as a forehead lift, to raise the brows. A brow lift improves the appearance of the forehead and the area around the eyes. A brow lift may be an appropriate procedure if the brows have become set lower and the eyes don't appear to fully open or if there are deep furrows between the brows giving a facial expression of anger.

Composite Facelift: A modern cosmetic surgical procedure that has been developed to improve the appearance of several areas of the face and neck. Unlike traditional facelift procedures that primarily stretched inelastic skin, the composite facelift also moves the underlying facial structures to achieve a natural and youthful appearance and yields a longer lasting result. Typically, the fat in the cheek pad is lifted and the muscles in the neck are tightened in addition to removal of inelastic skin.

"Crow's Feet": Wrinkles that appear at the outer corners of the eyes as people age. They typically appear deeper and more pronounced than wrinkles on other area of the face.

Elasticity: The ability of the skin to stretch and revert back to its original shape. As people age, the skin loses its elasticity and wrinkles commonly develop in the face and neck.

Endoscopic Surgery: Minimally invasive surgery where small incisions allow access to the area treated and a small camera on a fiber optics tube is used to guide the surgery.

Eyelid Surgery: Technically known as blepharoplasty, eyelid surgery is a cosmetic procedure that improves the appearance of the eyelids. Surgery can be performed on the upper lids, the lower lids, or on both.

Facelift: A facelift is a surgical procedure that improves the appearance of the face and neck, reducing visible signs of aging and restoring a more youthful appearance. Although facelifts were traditionally performed primarily by tightening excess skin that had lost elasticity, the modern standard of treatment is the composite facelift, where the underlying structures of the face and neck are moved to provide a more natural looking result.

F.A.C.S.: F.A.C.S. is an abbreviation that stands for Fellow of the American College of Surgeons.

Furrows: Wrinkles that develop in the forehead between the eyes that develop as people age. Furrows frequently give the facial expression of anger.

"Jowls": Sagging skin that develops below the chin or jaw line as the skin becomes thinner and less elastic as people age.

"Nip and Tuck": A traditional form of facelift procedure that primarily tightened excess skin on the face and neck that had lost its elasticity. This older type of facelift has generally been replaced with the more modern composite facelift technique.

"Waddle": Wrinkled, sagging skin on the neck caused by the skin becoming inelastic and the muscles in the neck becoming weakened with aging. This is typically corrected as part of a composite facelift procedure.

Notes

Notes

Notes

www.ingramcontent.com/pod-product-compliance
Ingram Content Group UK Ltd.
Pitfield, Milton Keynes, MK11 3LW, UK
UKHW062257290726
14090UKWH00017B/745